Tactical Density Training

Tactical Density Training

BY
Josh Bryant and Adam benShea

Tactical Density Training
JoshStrength, LLC and Adam benShea
Copyright © 2020
All rights reserved, including file sharing, the right to reproduce this work, in whole or any part, in any form. All inquiries must be directed to Josh Bryant and Adam benShea and have approval from both authors.

Table of Contents

Prologue vii
Introduction xi

Chapter I: Defining Density Training 1
Chapter II: Additional Benefits of Density Training 6
    Guiding Principles of the Program. 13
Chapter III: The Program. 29

Prologue
ByJosh Bryant

Bill "Kaz" Kazmaier was the best-built and most versatile super-heavyweight strength athlete of all time. A master of every strongman event, he supplemented his long list of talents with testicular fortitude. Overcoming some serious injuries, Kaz ran away with three *consecutive* World's Strongest Man championships, and was subsequently banned for being "too dominant."

Kaz epitomized the full package, harmonizing mind, body, and spirit. In a way, he was like a machine built decades before its time. Many iron game enthusiasts are only now realizing what a rare level of strength he possessed.

Kaz was no one-trick pony, either. Beyond his strongman adaptability, Kaz totaled 2,420 in powerlifting and was the first on the planet to bench-press 300 kilograms (661 pounds), well before souped-up super suits. Both records stood for decades (regardless of the weakening of judging standards and the introduction of strength assistance equipment).

Weighing in at 330 pounds while having a single-digit body fat percentage, Kaz was the all-around powerbuilding package!

When I was training for the 2005 Strongest Man in America contest, I talked weekly with Kaz. For hours, he would talk and I would listen. Like a sponge, I absorbed information.

In these conversations, Kaz repeatedly emphasized the importance of "busting out the stopwatch." This meant timing rest intervals between sets. Kaz believed that the biggest mistake trainees make is not tracking rest intervals. He said that this is why most strength athletes, and even bodybuilders, have piss-poor work capacities.

Prior to this, I did time my rest intervals between my compensatory acceleration training (CAT) sets of my main movements. After Kaz's urging, I started timing rest periods on everything, including assistance exercises.

The objective was not to just do more work; it was to do more work in the same amount of time, the same amount of work in less time, or even more work in less time. If I just did more without tracking time, I would never leave the gym, I could overtrain, and I might even enter a state of mental drudgery.

As I began to time everything, I added muscle and my waistline decreased (even as I ate Waffle House daily for breakfast, indulged in a lunch buffet, and capped the night off with a large pepperoni pizza).

Aside from the unintended aesthetic benefits, I easily ran away with victory at the five-event, same-day Strongest Man in America. In fact, I felt like I could have easily done the contest all over!

Fast-forward to 2006, when I decided to move to Texas to train at the world-famous Metroflex Gym. I became really serious about dropping body fat and getting jacked, so I trained under the tutelage of Metroflex owner Brian Dobson for a year. As our training volume went apeshit, the length of our workouts *never* increased. We watched the clock, as I watched my results skyrocket.

During this time period at Metroflex, I trained clients at the gym early in the morning until 10 a.m. Like an old cowboy Western movie, at high noon, Brian and I would hammer out our training session. In my two-hour break between work and working out, I would head a mile south on Cooper Street to the Starbucks inside Barnes and Noble. Along with loading up on a pre-workout caffeine jolt of coffee, I read books. One of these books was *Muscle Logic: Escalating Density Training* by Charles Staley. I was already very familiar with Staley's work from his time at ISSA, from whom I had earned my fitness certification.

I became even more interested in Staley's work when I read an intriguing quote by him on T Nation prior to reading his book: "When a biological system experiences a challenge, it modifies itself in order to be able to more easily meet similar challenges in the future." In other words, your muscles grow in proportion to the demands placed on them (assuming that your nutrition program is dialed in).

In this book, Staley did an absolutely beautiful job of laying out a cohesive, time-efficient system that with proper application would catalyze muscle hypertrophy, strength endurance and/or fat loss.

In fact, it reminded me of a story from our childhood…

Introduction

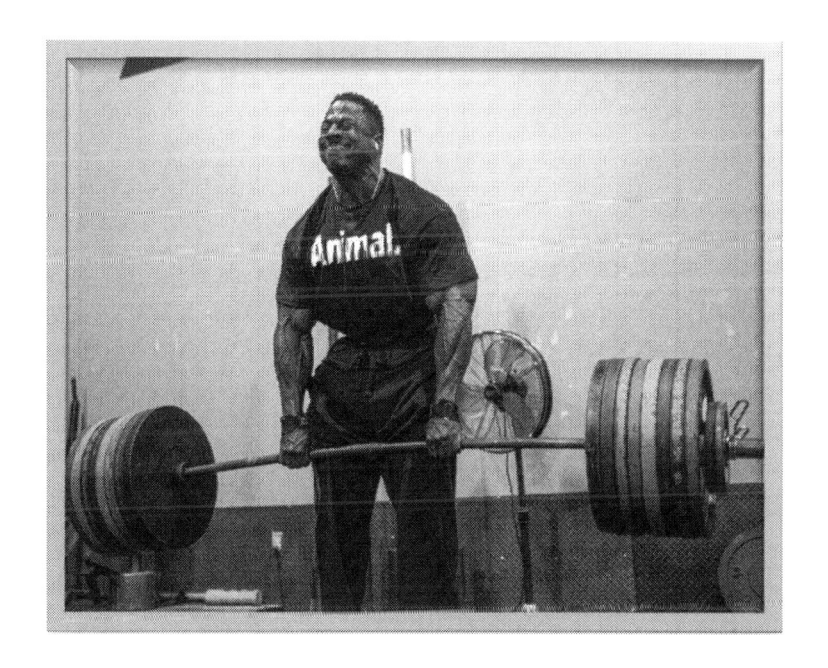

Joe Mackey

If you're already part of the Jailhouse Strong movement, you know the deal. If you're new to our books, welcome to the journey.

Our old gym provided us with a nexus of strength, mentorship, and learning. As you may remember from many of our earlier books, this gym also played host to a motley crew of ex-jocks, mystical strength gurus, old-time physical culturists, and tactical athletes. It was a target-rich environment for the flotsam and jetsam from the commercial gym environments, which like cubical culture slowly eats away at the raw and realistic human experience until all that remains are mindless sheep following the monotonous call for mind-numbing sensory overloading redundant behavior.

This gym was filled with individuals. One such character was Old School Frank. Everything about Frank was old-school.

We trained at this gym during the mid-1990s, so baggy pants and longer shorts were the norm. Old School Frank, however, would show up to workouts in high-cut athletic shorts, which broadcasted his massive and highly defined leg muscles. It was a time when most people wore their shirts untucked. Not Frank. His tank top was tucked so tightly into his shorts that his muscular six-pack was visible through the pulled fabric. He wore his socks high up to his knees, Michael Cooper style.

Old School Frank was a bodybuilder. But he was a throwback to the golden era of the sport. While many bodybuilders had that bloated, bulbous look, Frank's muscles were dense and proportional. Although muscle magazines and strip mall nutrition stores had started to push a potpourri of supplements "guaranteed" to get you strong, Frank's nutrition revolved around milk, eggs, salad, steak, and potatoes.

Old School Frank was a regular at the gym, and like many regulars, we sometimes talked. At this gym, conversations usually revolved around core topics like training, eating, and underground cage fighting in Old Mexico, while also floating into ancillary issues like dating advice and pyramid scheme marketing ideas.

So, when Frank showed up one day with a digital stopwatch around his neck, we felt comfortable opening up the conversation. This was no Flavor Flav of Public Enemy fashion statement. No, Frank was all about function over form.

"Hey Frank," we greeted him casually.

"Boys, how are you?" Frank responded, in his typical amicable way.

"All good. Hey, if you don't mind us asking, what's with the stopwatch? Are you doing some sprints outside today?"

"No," Frank said with a slight chuckle bubbling up from under his full, but well-trimmed manstache. "It's for the iron," he said with a thumb jerking back toward the dumbbell rack behind him.

"How so?" we asked with growing curiosity.

"Well, let's put it this way. You guys are familiar with the concept of progressive overload, right?"

We nodded in affirmation of familiarity with the concept which would later become a core pillar of our work with Jailhouse Strong.

"What does progressive overload mean to you?"

"Putting more weight on the bar," we answered, immediately remembering this pearl of wisdom from our powerlifting mentor Steve Holl.

"Absolutely, you've been talking with Big Steve, I see." Frank's face broke into a big smile at the mention of Steve's name. Steve had that effect on some folks. "But," Frank continued, "there is more to it than that. Yes, you want to add weight, incrementally. You also want to consider time. You fellas may not know this just yet. But time is powerful. It can be a terrible enemy or a great friend. It all depends on how you use it. Now, I use it as an ally."

As he said this, he struck his index finger into his massive chest as if to emphasize his personal agency in how he decides to use the powerful force of time.

"I look to get a little better every day. Each morning when you wake up, you have a choice. Will you regress or progress? Everything is in flux. Stagnation does not exist. Me? I choose to progress." His voice raised and took an intense tone as he settled into the brief lesson he was passing on to us.

"What does this mean for my training? I'll tell you. In the past, I settled for just adding weight. Now, I am turning it up a notch. I am timing my workouts, so I can complete the same amount of volume in less time. Or, on some days I lift more weights in the same amount of time. On the best days of training, I lift more weight in less time.

"This is how you get strong. This is how you develop muscular density. Now, boys, enough talk. It's a beautiful day. I'm going to train on the deck outside today."

Abruptly, "class" was over and Old School Frank walked to the outdoor training area. It was a beautiful day, with the sun shining.

Yeah, Frank was old-school alright.

But, we'll tell you something right now. When Frank took off his shirt to train, every girl in that gym stopped their workout to admire that classic torso. Like something envisioned by a sculptor of antiquity, Frank's build screamed unapologetic strength.

Sometimes, form follows function.

In the spirit of honoring those who influenced our density system, we heed the words of the great Bruce Lee, "Absorb what is useful, discard what is not, add what is uniquely your own."

We are sharing with you our own unique density system. Our advice is to follow it verbatim initially, and as you learn more about yourself and how you respond, you can alter it to make it uniquely your own.

We are providing you with two unique approaches: Gas Station Ready for tactical strength and conditioning and Chippendales Ready for the aesthetic minded.

Why It Works

Looking at muscle hypertrophy as the intended training goal, there are countless textbooks and numerous gurus who claim to have an ideal number of sets or reps for muscle growth. But, it's a little unclear. Some studies assert that really heavy weight with low reps catalyzes the most pronounced size increases, while others advocate higher reps and less weight. So which is it?

To further complicate matters, other studies claim that it's all about effort, regardless of the amount of weight lifted or the number of reps. That is, with enough intensity of effort, gains will ensue. And then some "lab coats" state that endless amounts of volume should be the focus (dismissing intensity and effort).

Some advocate very short rests to increase metabolic stress.

Some advocate rest-pauses.

Truthfully, we can say that none of these approaches are an infallible ticket to muscle-building salvation.

Many roads lead to the muscle-building Rome. However, rather than staying on the long, traditional paths, many folks look for shortcuts and detours to more efficiently reach their goals.

What we do know is the following: Intensity matters.

Anyone who tells you otherwise will also go on to tell you, "If your liver doesn't quiver and your bladder doesn't splatter, up the dose, it doesn't matter" (if you're not familiar with this old adage pushing for you to up your steroid dosage, you've had a wonderfully clean but perhaps uneventful training journey).

For aesthetics and size, strength is your base, and this has always been the case.

The recent chorus that sings otherwise is also pumping themselves full of pharmaceuticals. The late, legendary Bob Hoffman said, "Train for strength and shape will follow." He was right then and he is right now. Before the prevalence of drugs, every bodybuilder took this as gospel.

The bottom line is that strength is your base, and strength is built with high intensity and heavy weight.

Also, volume matters.

You can't just do a few heavy singles in a core lift and expect to maximize muscle hypertrophy; shoot, even for strength you will have to do more volume than this, along with corresponding accessory work. Training volume builds size and strength. Furthermore, the slower you gain size and strength, the more training volume you need.

Work Matters

Your muscles rapidly adapt to the work they are asked to do. So, the played-out 1990s Muscle and Fitness routine may produce some initial results, but those gains will plateau quickly.

Why?

Well, if you routinely train with 20-pound dumbbells but never increase poundage, your muscles will become just strong enough to lift the 20-pound dumbbell, but not more than that. Muscles grow only enough to stay in line with the demands placed on them. Take a look outside of the gym. A manual laborer may acquire a level of strength. Yet, they will lift only the amount of weight their job routinely demands. While the laborer may have muscle endurance specific to their task, they do not continually overload their muscles or do more work (unless they are chasing some overtime). Furthermore, they do not condense the amount of time in which they perform the same amount of work (unless they have a "helicopter boss"). In fact, as technology improves, oftentimes the laborer may do less physical work. If that same laborer moves into a managerial position, their work might become even less physically demanding. As a result, they watch their size and strength decrease.

The muscles of these laborers are big enough and just strong enough to do the work asked of them and no more.

The way to get bigger and stronger is by doing more work.

What do we mean by work?

Work is not getting all "crunk" (that is, excited and full of energy) to get your "instamotivation" deadlift workout on fleek. Work is an actual real, measurable equation.

The Work formula is Mass x Distance (M x D = W).

Muscle grows and strength increases, in a large part, in proportion to the amount of work you do (assuming the weight is heavy enough, the reps are quality, and you do not overtrain). All of this is handled by following the program we lay out.

Simply, the density progression ensures you do more work as time goes on. But, for work to be effective, it must be within a time frame that does not just drag on. What good is 10 sets of bench press over four hours if you previously did eight sets with the same weight in 30 minutes? Work must increase, but your workout time can't keep increasing.

Chapter I: Defining Density Training

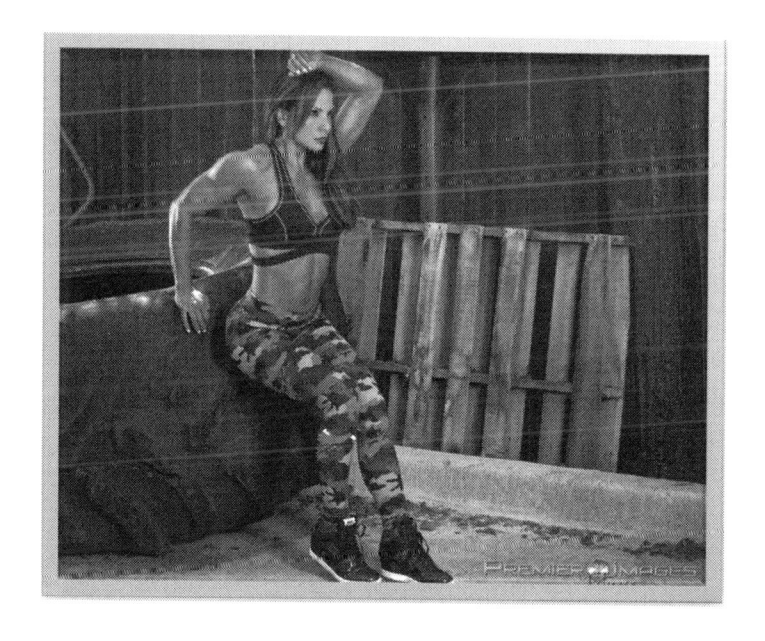

Priscilla Smith

BASIC MEANS FUNDAMENTAL, not elementary.
Density is about as basic as it gets.
Density is not mystical; It simply looks at training volume and duration. Training volume is the workload that combines

the sets x reps x weight. OG, Old School, Golden Era bodybuilder Chuck Sipes pioneered this concept as a measurable metric. He called it tonnage.

In honor of the great Sipes, we will refer to training volume as tonnage. Duration is the length of time it takes to execute an exercise, multiple exercises paired together, or an entire training session.

So, your training density is simply the amount of tonnage you complete in a specified exercise, or training session, inside of a specific duration.

Now there are professional athletes, with unlimited time to train, who split up their training into multiple sessions a day. However, with work and family commitments, most folks do not have the luxury to train multiple times a day. With this in mind, the only way to continually put in more work without creating marathon training sessions or having to train multiple times a day is to increase density.

How do we do that?

Past Examples

Density training is not a new concept within the Jailhouse Strong movement. Below are some past examples we have used.

Total Repetition Method: This method may be used with any type of strength training exercise.

All it means is the chosen exercise is performed in the fewest number of sets to hit the prescribed number of repetitions. Using the total repetition method, 100 pull-ups might look something like this: *Set 1 – 15 reps, Set 2 – 12 reps, Set 3 – 11 reps, Set 4 – 10 reps, Set 5 – 10 reps, Set 6 – 9 reps, Set 7 – 8 reps, Set 8 – 7 reps, Set 9 – 7 reps, Set 10 – 6 reps, Set 11 – 5 reps.*

This would be progressed by doing more total reps in the same amount of time or doing the same number of reps in less time after establishing a baseline. Either progression method makes the program denser.

Because of the success of our total repetition program, it plays a vital role in our density program.

The Juarez Valley Method: This method consists of ascending and descending repetitions in an alternating fashion. The repetitions are performed in descending order on all odd-numbered sets, and on even-numbered sets, reps are performed in ascending order until they finally meet in the middle.

A Juarez Valley 20 looks like this:

    Set 1:   20 reps
    Set 2:   1 rep
    Set 3:   19 reps
    Set 4:   2 reps
    Set 5:   18 reps
    Set 6:   3 reps
    Set 7:   17 reps
    Set 8:   4 reps
    Set 9:   16 reps
    Set 10: 5 reps
    Set 11: 15 reps
    Set 12: 6 reps
    Set 13: 14 reps
    Set 14: 7 reps
    Set 15: 13 reps
    Set 16: 8 reps
    Set 17: 12 reps
    Set 18: 9 reps

Set 19: 11 reps
Set 20: 10 reps

Between each set, walk eight feet across your "cell" (keeping in the spirit that this routine evolved out of the penitentiary in Old Mexico).

This method could be done with any movement from push-ups to lunges.

Progression is achieved by doing more total reps in the same amount of time or doing the same number of reps in less time (after establishing a baseline). Either progression method makes the program denser.

Other past examples from some of our previous books include the Jailhouse Method, rest-pause sets, the 8 x 8 program, and all of our cluster set variations. The possibilities are endless. As you will see, we have built on and fine-tuned the density progressions from our previous works.

Set Duration/More Work

Let's develop the way in which density training works inside of a routine.

For example, suppose you are following a modified German volume training program and you squat 10 sets of six reps with 300 pounds. You complete all 10 sets in 30 minutes. That is 60 total reps with 300 pounds in 30 minutes. If next week you do 10 sets of seven reps in 30 minutes, you have increased your training tonnage. Assuming you do not drop below 300 pounds (which we do not allow) in the program, your training tonnage has increased. As long as you complete more than 60 reps with 300 pounds in 30 minutes, your tonnage has increased and therefore your density has increased. 300 pounds x 60 reps is 18,000 pounds of training tonnage. If we increase your working weight to 315 pounds, we have increased your training tonnage to 18,900. Assuming this is completed in 30 minutes, you have increased your training density.

Training density with the same workout duration can be increased by adding more weight, doing more reps, and/or doing more sets.

The reason we do not drop weight for a tonnage measurement is as follows. If you squatted 100 pounds for 10 sets of 20 reps, your tonnage would equate to 20,000 pounds. At best, this would offer a muscle endurance effect, in contrast to the highly anabolic 10 sets of six reps with 300 pounds. SO MAKE SURE TO FOLLOW THE INSTRUCTIONS!

Decreased Duration/Set Work

Let's stick with our hypothetical modified German volume plan of 10 sets of six reps on squats with 300 pounds executed in 30 minutes (mentioned above). If we tell you now that you must complete that load in 24 minutes, you are now completing 18,000 pounds of training tonnage in 20 percent less time. If you do the same amount of training tonnage in a reduced amount of time, you have increased training density.

Set Duration/Set Work/New Exercise

In our version of density training, we do include supersets. However, they include a primary exercise and a secondary exercise. For instance, with the modified German volume training example, you are completing 10 sets of six reps in 30 minutes in the squat with 300 pounds. Each set of squats is supersetted with four reps of leg curls.

Chapter II: Additional Benefits of Density Training

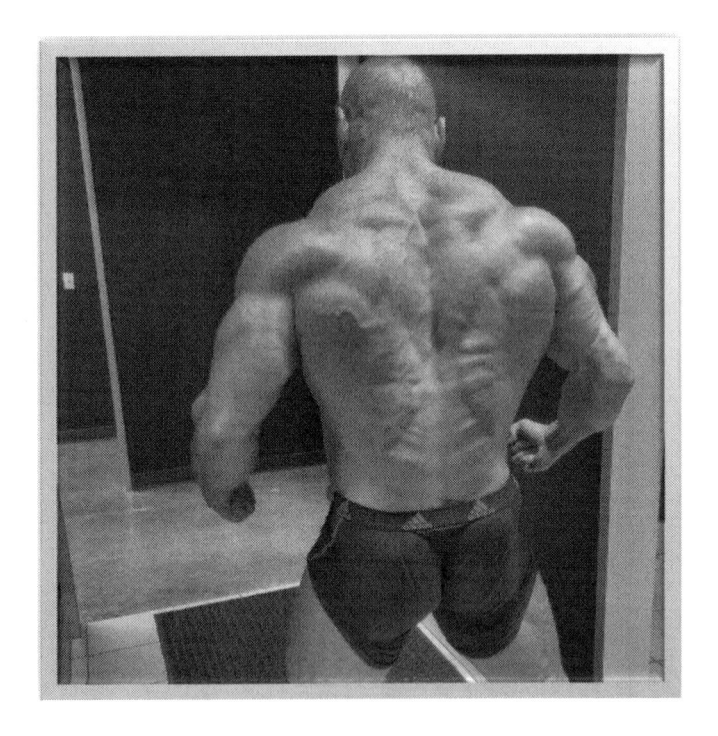

Ed Brown

Dialogue is important. Through verbal communication, ideas are exchanged, advice is imparted, and lessons are taught.

While some conversations are petty, superficial, and forgettable, the ones we shared in our youth with our fellow gym dwellers were deep, insightful, and unforgettable. We learned so much about the pitfalls of dating cabaret dancers, the benefits of a well-planned barfight strategy, and unorthodox but effective approaches to training.

Fortunately, we were able to have many of these valuable exchanges. The older lifters provided guidance. We listened and remembered.

However, not everyone at our gym took the time to talk. Big Bob never seemed to have time. Broad in chest, back, and shoulders, Bob was hard to miss. We'd see him training at a frantic pace around the dumbbell rack. Sometimes, we'd catch a glimpse of him around town, looking polished in a pinstriped suit. Although he had the build of a turn-of-the-century strongman, Bob was an investment banker, and he dressed the part. He also acted the part, always too busy to talk.

So, when we saw Big Bob training with Old School Frank, we didn't expect conversation. However, just as he was finishing up his workout, Bob waved us over.

"Hey fellas, got a second?" Bob asked while briskly wiping his sweat-drenched face with a hand towel.

It seemed odd for Bob to ask whether we had time, when he seemed to be the one who was always rushing everywhere. Clearly, he respected time.

"Yes," we answered with a nod and more than a little curiosity as to why he picked this moment to talk with us.

"Frank here told me that he told you guys a little about his training methods," Bob said with a tilt of his head in the direction of Old School Frank. "He said you guys were alright. You knew how to listen. I respect that, people who listen. There seems to be less of that these days. People want to open their mouths, even when nothing thoughtful comes out.

"You know, nobody ever lost anything by listening. But, hey, I'll tell you plenty of folks have lost plenty just by speaking. So, I respect when people, like you guys, listen. It's getting rare, especially among the young. I wish they knew how much they could learn just by listening.

"Along with that, and I'll keep it brief…I don't want to keep you, I respect time. You know, I've made a lot of money. The thing is I know I can make more. I will make more.

"Time"—at the mention of that word, one that was clearly loaded with significance to him, Bob looked out the open warehouse door of the gym—"is different. I trade commodities. But time is the most precious commodity there is. The more time you get, the less of it you have.

"Young people may not understand that as much as older folks, but that doesn't make it any less true."

Bob had our rapt attention, so we stood in silence waiting to hear what else he had to share.

"Right," Bob nodded in affirmation and appreciation for our silence, "that's why I like this type of training that Frank put together. You know that he's real selective about who he trains. Actually, he only agreed to work with me because I throw in some blue-chip stock tips as part of our exchange.

"Anyway, this program Frank put together, the one he was telling you about the other day, it's great. First and foremost, it makes the most of my time in the gym; it is time efficient. I'm moving the whole time. I stay warm and ready. I come to the gym with a focused intent to move more weight on the bar and lift it in less time. Whether in the boardroom or the bedroom, you want a clear intention."

At that, he gave us a quick smile. Bob was known around town as a bit of a ladies' man, maybe even a lothario.

"You know what else?" Bob's voice was speeding up, as he was clearly excited about this training program. "This type of workout has auto-regulation. On the days when I'm really feeling it, I can go hog wild. You can't shackle success. You gotta give a hero some room to shake off the fetters of mediocrity.

"Also, I've dropped some pounds. I'll be looking good when I take my boat down to the Dry Tortugas next month."

At that, Bob checked the time on his Rolex Yacht Master.

"Alright, I got to run. I have a lunch meeting in 15 minutes. Good talk."

We considered asking him about the stick tips, but he was off to the locker room before we could get our question out. We were left with some wisdom that we still remember today.

Here are some reasons why training density can benefit your training, or the training of your clients.

Time Efficiency. The benefit of additional training volume quickly dissipates when training sessions drag on for endless hours. Regardless of the physiological benefits, time is non-refundable. Time is the most precious commodity we have. Unlike just about everything else, the more time you receive, the less of it you have. So, use time wisely. If something can be done in less time without sacrificing the benefits, well, it simply just makes sense.

Progressive Overload. Since we continually increase the load in volume and intensity over time, your body will adapt to it. As your numbers improve, you will become bigger, broader, and stronger without having to continually spend more time in the gym. Volume is extremely important for muscle growth and strength. When you continually increase the amount of training tonnage, assuming diet is in check, your muscles will grow and you will get stronger.

Fat Loss. Even now, in the "roaring fitness 20s," the old adage of move more and eat less remains true for fat loss. So, you have a choice: Start implementing testosterone-ridding jogs that leave you physically flaccid and mentally unfulfilled or opt for our proven density training that greatly increases the "move more variable" in an interval style and releases a cascade of anabolic hormones that will expedite the fat loss process while packing on slabs of muscle.

Auto-Regulation. This simply means that when you feel good, go for it, come out guns a blazing. Conversely, when you feel off, pull back. With density training, you are not boxed in with specific rep schemes and exact rest intervals. When you feel good, you can do more reps. When you feel off, do less. You can adjust to how you feel on that day. With our density program, you have one objective: do more work than you did last time.

Increased Work Capacity. When you improve the amount of volume you are able to complete in a specific duration, you have effectively increased your physical preparedness or your ability to do work. In fact, this is why this program is very effective for off-season powerlifting; a major objective for any serious powerlifter should be increased work capacity. Improved work capacity and strength endurance not only are effective for immediately increasing muscle hypertrophy, fat loss, and strength, but also help you down the road. Greater work capacity serves as a proper volume base, upon which you taper according to the specific demands of a particular powerlifting meet or strength event. Moreover, when you maintain your strength while doing an endurance block of training, you will have the ability to maximize the work necessary for maximal hypertrophy or special ops training.

No Bullshit Progressions. We live in very strange times. While broke financial advisors distribute money management wisdom, we remember the witticism of our friend and mentor, the late Strength Sensei Charles Poliquin, who reminded us: Don't trust a virgin sex therapist. In a time when so many Internet con artists and self-appointed social media messiahs want to turn abstract beliefs into concrete "science" and morph facts into metaphysical meanderings, it's easy to forget about real, measurable results that go beyond a feel-good circle jerk. We are looking at training tonnage and the time you take to complete the training sessions. Numbers don't lie. Either you are making progress or you're not.

Temperature. If you train outside of a perfect, climate-controlled facility, listen up! Whether you're training on an isolated frozen tundra or in a local YMCA that just doesn't seem to be able to balance climate control, you are going to have to stay moving between sets to feel warm and ready to go. With the constant movement of density training, your core temperature stays up and you stay ready to go. This is valuable not only to the power and speed athlete but also for the athlete battling Father Time by fighting another day to maintain health and stay ready.

Concentration. Where attention goes, energy flows. Idle time is the devil's playhouse! Often, when prolonged rest periods are advocated, athletes start bird-dogging the toned bodies in spandex, scrolling through social media on their phones, or talking with some gym denizens about the new supplement line. All of these behaviors destroy the mental training zone.

The purpose of training is not to socialize or pick up a date. However, it should be noted that if your goal is to find some sort of a relationship (physical, romantic, emotional, or whatever), take a cue from the independent film *The Tao of Steve*. Do something excellent in their presence. Make the training facility your element, your place to broadcast your excellence. Focus on your training, be excellent, and win the heart (at least for the night) of your gym crush.

Cluster Set Benefit. Cluster sets are those in which the main sets are broken into several parts. For example, instead of doing a set of nine straight reps, you do a set of 3+3+3 reps, which allows for a very short rest period within the set. That intraset rest period allows you to lift more total weight than you'd be able to with straight reps. This provides a greater anabolic stimulus.

Clear Intention. Okay, you are in Bangalore, India, and you head out for a night on the town to Chin Lung Resto Bar, where you go out to grab a shot of Old Monk, washed down with a cold Kingfisher, and maybe even sing some karaoke. Your clear intention is to verify that Kingfisher really is the king of good times. In the weight room you need the same focus, or clear intention. When your goal is to do more tonnage in the same duration or the same amount of tonnage in a shorter time, you have a clear-cut intention; as Napoleon Hill would say, you possess a definitiveness of purpose. You have a defined goal to accomplish on a specific day, in a set amount of time. With this in mind, we marry the east and the west—the eastern concept of intentionality and the western one of a measurable goal—for a harmonious union.

Technique Enhancement. By working movements, and stopping shy of true failure and technique degradation, the athlete is forced to focus on technique and enhance motor learning patterns.

Excitement. With our system, athletes are able to perpetually break their own personal records. Assuming you're adequately resting and properly eating, you will be able to break your own records for a long time coming. No sweeter victory than victory over self. Or, as Plato wrote: "The first and greatest victory is to conquer yourself."

Guiding Principles of the Program

As you progress through this program, here are some important principles to use as navigational points. They'll help you better understand the program and customize it for your particular needs.

Avoid Failure

We are after total tonnage here. So, if you fail early on, subsequent sets will suffer. Make an effort to enhance your technique on all lifts, but especially on major compound lifts. You want to display the skill of strength with technical mastery. Think total tonnage, not "rep records."

Stay within Rep Ranges

Rep ranges are specifically there for a reason. This is for technique enhancement and to avoid fatigue early on.

Pair Exercises with Non-Competing Muscle Groups

Pairing a Hercules chin-up and biceps curl causes a very taxing localized fatigue to the elbow flexors, and there is a time and a place for this aesthetic-based training. However, with our density training, we are looking to create a more "globalized" fatigue, rather than an isolated one. So, Hercules chin-ups would be paired with dips, triceps extensions with hammer curls, and overhead presses with lat pulldowns. We want to create a greater degree of systemic fatigue by pairing exercises that do not hinder each other.

More on Antagonistic Pairing

Agonist muscles, or prime mover muscles, cause a move to happen through their own activation. For example, as you lock out a bench press, your triceps contract to extend your elbows. The antagonist muscles operate in the opposite fashion. Some people think of it as the agonist muscles have the agony of doing all the work, although anyone familiar with hard training knows that "agony" in a workout becomes a blessing for muscle growth.

Antagonistic muscles work in synergy: **When one of the muscles contracts, the other relaxes.** Sticking with the triceps example, when the triceps contract, the opposing biceps relax; if they didn't, you wouldn't lock out the barbell and your muscles would be in an isometric stalemate. This is part of the reason why advanced lifters and athletes can produce more force; through executing a motor pattern properly, they have trained antagonistic muscles to relax sooner and more abruptly through a process called reciprocal inhibition.

In bodybuilding, supersetting often describes alternating two exercises for the same body part. Historically, however, supersetting is pairing two antagonistic movements alternately performed, and each movement is repeated alternately for the required number of reps; we will stick with the traditional meaning.

For example, bench presses and seal rows would be a superset.

Science Speaks

Many studies confirm the efficacy of supersets. Let's look at two that were eye-opening studies that broadened our horizons on this topic, while maintaining context.

A 2009 study published in the *Journal of Sports Sciences* entitled "Effects of agonist-antagonist complex resistance training on upper body strength and power development" demonstrated the efficiency of supersets. Over the course of eight weeks, a group that trained the bench press with bench pulls (an opposing pulling movement for the upper back) improved bench press strength slightly over a group that trained the bench press with traditional sets.

Although the superset training group did not have a statistically significant surge in bench press strength over the control group, the study did demonstrate the efficiency of superset training: The same amount of work could basically be done in half the time without compromising strength gains. So, if nothing else, superset training is an effective means of cutting down time in the gym and making gains.

A 2005 study published in the *Journal of Strength and Conditioning Research* entitled "Acute effect on power output of alternating an agonist and antagonist muscle exercise during complex training" implied that not only does superset training save time, but it hypothetically enhances power.

The study found that rugby players with strength-training experience increased power by 4.7 percent when training the bench press throw in a complex, as opposed to doing the bench press throw alone.

Science says we will save time and not sacrifice strength and power gains from workouts and, quite possibly, even enhance them.

The Lab Meets the Real World

It is important to note that a minority of advanced strength athletes train this way. The subjects in the aforementioned studies were not competitive lifters. We believe this is because of fatigue and drainage of psychic energy through focused intention.

Strength is a product of the central nervous system (CNS) because strength athletes have very efficient motor recruitment patterns. So, in lay terms, they are so skilled at the movements they perform that they fatigue faster. Studies have shown the stronger an individual is, the longer rest intervals need to be between sets. Remember, we are talking about trained strength athletes, not the dude with a couple veins in his biceps at LA Fitness who does ring pull-ups and Turkish get-ups to assist his golf game.

While there are some elite athletes who do not use paired sets, every strength athlete, functional training athlete, and tactical athlete can benefit from a modified type of superset training. We call our density approach to superset training the Tactical Density Training (TDT).

This program focuses on pairing agonist and antagonist muscles together. This is where you will start for the program. Along with managing fatigue, this keeps you focused with intention on the primary exercise you are executing.

Here it is, where the rubber hits the road.

YOU WILL HAVE A PRIMARY AND A SECONDARY FOCUS.

Here is an example. If you are capable of doing a 200-pound overhead press (OHP) max and a pull-up max with 120 pounds over your bodyweight, an example of emphasizing OHP looks like this in Tactical Density Training:

Set 1 TDT
>OHP 160 Pounds × 5 Reps—Pull-Ups Bodyweight × 5 reps

Set 2 TDT
>OHP 160 Pounds × 4 Reps—Pull-Ups Bodyweight × 5 reps

Set 3 TDT
>OHP 160 Pounds × 3 Reps—Pull-Ups Bodyweight × 5 reps

The inverse of TDT placing the emphasis on the upper back would look like this:

Set 1 TDT
>Pull-Up 80 Pounds Over Bodyweight × 6 Reps—OHP 110x8

Set 2 TDT
>Pull-Up 80 Pounds Over Bodyweight × 5 Reps—OHP 110x8

Set 3 TDT
>Pull-Up 80 Pounds Over Bodyweight × 5 Reps—OHP 110x8

In the words of Lee Haney, "stimulate not annihilate" is the objective of the antagonist muscle.

With TDT and alternating exercises back and forth in the manner described, you will do two things. First, it will ensure that the blood supply is limited to a relatively small area, rather than up and down your entire body. This assists speedy recovery of the targeted muscle while the antagonist is working, and vice versa.

Alternatively, by exercising the muscles on both sides of the joint(s), normal flexibility and function will be maintained.

Here are some examples of antagonistic pairs

- Abductor/Adductor
- Biceps/Triceps
- Pectoral/Latissimus
- Quadriceps/Hamstrings
- Upper Back/Chest

If this is confusing, you can also think of opposing movement patterns. Some examples are:

- Bench Press/Seal Row
- Leg Extension/Leg Curl
- Overhead Press/Pull-Up
- Hip Abduction/Hip Adduction
- Biceps Curl/Triceps Extension

Some things require clarification; for example, in a true, full-body movement like a farmer's walk, we will guide you and include something that will help you, but not sacrifice the primary movement (in the tradition of Joe Weider's staggered set principle).

Superset Cautions

Whether it's Tactical Density Training or any other program involving supersets, we advise you to really take into account the demands placed on the lower back. On the surface, an Olympic pause squat and a Romanian deadlift seem like a logical pair, but both place a very high demand on the lower back. In this case, a much smarter choice would be a leg curl.

Keeping with the lower back theme, when you are executing pressing movements, make sure that opposing row movements do not expose the lower back. For example, if you are focusing on the bench press, regardless of what the lab coats in the NSCA text say, do not superset bent rows. For many, they cause a greater amount of low back stress compared to even a regular deadlift. Opt for a seal row!

Weight Lifting Intensity Levels

When you read over the program, you will notice that some of the weights and reps are listed as RPE with a corresponding number. **RPE**, in strength training, is the **rate of perceived exertion**. It's a subjective measurement of the difficulty of a set.

Decades ago, the RPE scale was introduced by a Swedish researcher, the late Gunnar Borg, as a measurement of fatigue on a scale of 6 to 20. Since then, powerlifters like Mike Tuchscherer and others have used RPEs with a more simplified scale and as a way to self-regulate intensity. For example, a strength coach may assign athletes training sessions without specific weights or percentages, but just ask them to work up to a corresponding RPE or ask them to rate how difficult a set is using an RPE.

There is no standardized RPE scale for strength training; Borg's original was geared more toward endurance activities. Our scale is listed below. When we assign an RPE, it means the following:

RPE	Meaning
4	Light weight for active recovery or mobility
5	Warm-up weight
6	Too light to have a significant training effect
7	Could have performed an additional three to five reps at the end of the set
8	Could have performed two or three additional reps at the end of the set
9	Could have performed one additional rep at the end of the set, maybe two
10	At a max, no additional reps could be performed at the end of the set

A majority of weights in the major lifts will be clearly assigned with the exact poundage. However, on smaller and secondary movements, we will use this scale, so please familiarize yourself with it.

Fast Gainers/Slow Gainers

One of the most important concepts we were introduced to, directly from the late, legendary Dr. Fred Hatfield, is the difference between fast gainers and slow gainers.

"Fast gainers" are people who gain size and strength the easiest. Certain training patterns separate the two categories. For example, fast gainers are oftentimes able to do only 4 to 6 reps at 80 percent of their one-rep max on a given day, while lifters who have trouble making gains are able to rep out at around 15 to 20 reps with 80 percent of their max.

Fast gainers will frequently have poor anaerobic strength endurance. This is explainable, in part, by the fact that their muscular structure is probably mostly white muscle fiber, which has fast – twitch/low-oxidative capabilities. Conversely, slow gainers probably have mostly red muscle fiber or slow-twitch fibers that are more suited for endurance and therefore may possess greater ability for rapid recovery during a set.

Fast/Slow Gainer Adjustments

Most people who train seriously are more to the faster gainer side. It is human nature to engage in activities toward which one has a natural propensity. Even weightlifting "hard gainers" are oftentimes really easy gainers, compared to the public at large.

If you are a hard gainer, someone who does 15 reps or more at 80 percent of your one-rep max, you can make the following adjustments:

- Increase RPE by 1, so a 7 becomes an 8.
- Increase the number of allowable reps in a set by 50%, so if it is a max of 6 reps, you can do 9, for example.
- Increase the amount of allowable reps in a quarter by 50%, so if it's 50 reps, you will do 75.
- Shorten your training week from 7 days to 5 or 6 days.

For the fast gainers, those of you doing six reps or fewer at 80 percent of your one-rep max, you can make the following adjustments:

- Extend the work week to 9 days (add extra rest or activity recovery days).
- Decrease the number of allowable reps in a set by one, so if it is a max of 6 reps, you can do 5, for example.

- Decrease the amount of allowable reps in a quarter by 25%, so if it's 40 reps, you will do 30.

A vast majority of readers will not fall into either extreme camp and should complete the program as prescribed.

Warming Up

Charles Poliquin said it best: If your warm-up takes longer than your workout, you are a "twatwaffle"; nonetheless, it is still important to do a proper warm-up.

Having over 40 years of combined paid coaching experience in the fitness industry between the two of us, we have seen it all. That includes twatwaffles hogging a platform at the gym to foam roll for an hour as they complain about their decreasing stock portfolio to their personal trainer while trying to line up a night on the town with their co-worker's old lady on social media.

Of course, there is the complete opposite approach to warm-ups, exhibited by that alcoholic high school coach with a 60-inch waist, who proudly preached his beliefs that if every grown man took a combination of Dianabol and Xanax, the national debt would be erased. Anyway, this dude would not let the kids warm up. Apparently, between swigs of Jack Daniels, he read scientific journals that said warm-ups were not necessary, and no one starting off with 450 on squat "had died yet."

We take the middle ground, like Poliquin, realizing warm-ups are important but should not take the length of a training session.

Warming up is an art. If you do not have a routine, start with our suggested one and hone it to your needs.

Some of the benefits of a proper warm-up:

- IMPROVED PERFORMANCE!
- Increased muscle contraction and relaxation speed
- More "economical"/efficient movement patterns
- Reduced muscle stiffness
- Improved oxygen utilization
- Improved motor unit recruitment for all-out activity (i.e., more coordinated movements with increased intensity)
- Increased blood flow
- Brings the heart rate to the proper level for beginning exercise
- Increases mental focus for the task at hand, be it intervals or competition, by an increased "arousal," or enthusiasm, eagerness, and mental readiness

General Warm-Up

Now, if you are looking for an in-depth scientific analysis on why it's important to warm up, corner a doctor at your next cocktail party or plow through WebMD online. In the meantime, we will take you through a cursory look at the benefits of warming up and, more importantly, how to warm up.

Dynamic stretching will be the major piece of the warm-up pie. Many folks are successful jumping immediately into our dynamic stretching routine by starting at half speed and gradually working up to full speed. However, we recommend that you start with a general warm-up before beginning a dynamic stretch.

The general warm-up takes two to five minutes and should be something to elevate your body temperature. It could be an easy jog, a brisk walk, or your favorite cardio machine (if you train at a gym). Finally, after you complete the general warm-up, proceed to the dynamic stretching routine.

What about static stretching?

We recommend that you conduct all static stretching and proprioceptive neuromuscular facilitation (PNF) stretching routines *after* your workout, not before. Static stretching prior to workouts can take away from explosivity and strength. Of course, there are some folks who have performed these workouts with great success after beginning with static stretching.

Dynamic Stretching

Dynamic stretching incorporates active (meaning you actively stretch without outside assistance) range of motion (ROM). Dynamic stretches generally look somewhat like sport-specific or training-specific motions. Unlike static stretching, dynamic stretches are not held at the end of the range of motion.

A plethora of patterns can be utilized. It's important to remember that movements similar to those you will be training will provide you with the greatest benefit. Unless you enjoy being on the injured reserve list, when you're stretching dynamically, pay attention to not exceed the currently established range of motion for the joint(s) being stretched.

There are two important details to keep in mind to maximize benefit and minimize risk. First, establish an even, controlled rhythm, with all movements initially well within the current range of motion. Then, gradually increase the amplitude of the movement until you are at the desired level of tension at the end point of the movement.

Remember, these are specialized movements and care must be taken with their use. Make it a habit to precede dynamic stretching with a general warm-up of two to five minutes.

To reiterate: We recommend not stretching a cold muscle!

Warm-Up
The following is an example of a warm-up for an intense workout.

- 2- to 5-minute brisk walk warm-up
- Dynamic stretching
- Walk on toes—2 sets of 15 yards
- Walk on heels—2 sets of 15 yards
- Arm swings—2 sets of 10 clockwise and counterclockwise
- Arm hugs—2 sets of 10 reps
- Straight leg kicks—3 sets of 15 yards
- Leg swings—2 sets of 15 reps
- High knees—3 sets of 15 yards
- Walking lunges—3 sets of 15 yards
- Lateral lunges—2 sets of 10 reps (back and forth, do not hold end position)
- Wrist sways—3 sets of 15 each way
- Hula hip swings—2 sets of 10 clockwise and counterclockwise

Upon completing this warm-up, start warming up for the first lifting movement of the day. To see visual examples of dynamic warm-ups, please turn to the Jailhouse Strong YouTube channel.

Warm-Up Weights
As we've discussed, the benefits of a proper warm-up are well documented. Some of the innumerable benefits include

more efficient movement patterns and increased mental readiness. Your muscles and joints also get primed. No successful lifter today forgoes this critical step. Why should you?

The warm-up moves in a funnel fashion from general to specific. After the general warm-up and dynamic stretching, you move to the specific phase. So, upon completion of the warm-up described above, if you're squatting, continue your warm-up by squatting. Use this same logic for deadlifts and bench presses—or any lift, for that matter. Warming up in a specific manner will get you mentally and physically ready to dominate the training session.

An added benefit of doing warm-ups is additional volume. Volume equals weight x sets x reps, so squatting progressively heavier submaximal weights for 3 sets of 5 reps (none even close to straining) adds significantly extra training volume without adding extra time to your training session. Strength is a skill; this skill is enhanced with a specific warm-up.

Here are a few examples of warm-ups for the first movement of the day:

Squats

- 45 x 6 x 4 sets
- 95 x 5 x 2 sets
- 135 x 4
- 165 x 3
- 195 x 2
- 225 x 1
- 255 (work set)

Bench Press

- 45 x 6 x 4 sets
- 135 x 6 x 2 sets
- 225 x 6
- 275 x 2
- 315 x 1
- 350 x 1
- 375 (work set)

Deadlifts

- 45 x 6 x 4 sets
- 135 x 3 x 3 sets
- 225 x 2 x 2 sets
- 275 x 1
- 315 x 1
- 365 x 1
- 405 (work set)

After you have warmed up and executed the work sets of the first movement "quarter" in the program (more about that in the next chapter), you are ready to jump into the second quarter. We recommend one warm-up set with a submaximal weight for each accessory movement, just to familiarize yourself with the movement pattern you will be performing.

Final Thoughts on Warm-Up

Keep in mind that this warm-up is a good starting point, but you actively form it to what works best for you and what will get you warm for the activities at hand.

While the need to warm up is validated by many scientific studies, the individual approach to the warm-up is an art. The longer you train and practice, the better artist you become.

Finally, before you put intervals into practice, we highly recommend you do the activity at a submaximal pace for a couple of test runs before going all out.

Warm up to maximize results and minimize risks!

Chapter III: The Program

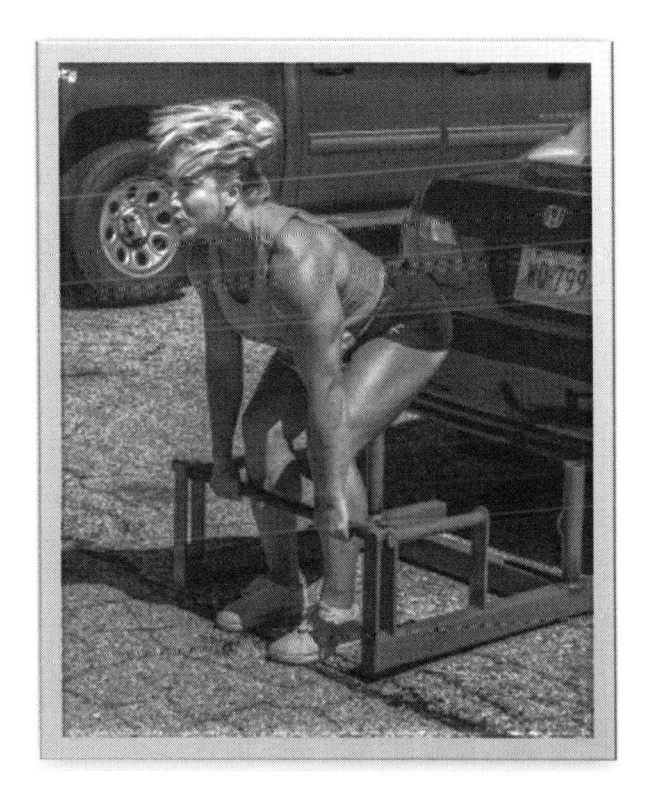

Britanny Diamond

This program is divided into four quarters, just like a football game. Each quarter is symbolic.

Tactical Density Training

First quarter, come charging out of the tunnel. This is where you set the pace for the training session. Like this old, heavy-set Chicano told both of us before our respective boxing matches, down the street from the infamous "Las Conchas" bar, draw first blood. The first quarter sets the tone to build unstoppable snow-balling momentum. This quarter lasts for 15 minutes and has the objective of completing 50 reps within the time frame.

Second quarter, the objective is to "keep on keeping on," in the words of Joe Dirt (and Curtis Mayfield before him). You should be adding to the momentum you have built. But, if the first quarter did not go as planned, this is your chance to get the game on track. It ain't over until the fat lady sings, and she hasn't even shown up to the stadium yet because the game is not yet halfway over. This quarter lasts 12 minutes and has the objective of completing 40 reps within the time frame.

Up next, the third quarter. It is easy for a football player, in the third quarter, to forget why he is in the game. The work has been so difficult and he is so focused on taking care of his responsibilities, he often forgets the love of the game and why he started playing in the first place. If you are having a great session, don't gloat. Stay focused while having fun; remember, you started training because you love it. If things have not been going your way, have a short memory and focus on what you are doing right here and now, and the love you have for it. This quarter lasts eight minutes and has the objective of completing 35 reps within the time frame.

The fourth quarter is where you play up. Odds are that this session has been a dogfight! But, now it's fourth and goal. Finish strong. Punch it! Even if you are losing, make the opposing team keep in their starters. Don't go belly-up and give the scrubs a chance to play. They get splinters in their ass from riding the pine for a reason. They do not belong on the field of play with you. This quarter lasts eight minutes and has the objective of completing 30 reps within the time frame.

Further Instructions
Quarter 1: On the primary movement (the one listed first), start with a weight with which you can do 10 to 12 reps; the objective is to complete 50 reps within 15 minutes. For the secondary exercises, the prescribed number of reps and the corresponding targeted RPE/intensity level is listed.

Quarter 2: On the primary movement (the one listed first), start with a weight with which you can do 12 to15 reps; the objective is to complete 40 reps within 12 minutes. For the secondary exercises, the prescribed number of reps and the corresponding targeted RPE/intensity level is listed.

Quarter 3: On the primary movement (the one listed first), start with a weight with which you can do 12 to15 reps; the objective is to complete 35 reps within eight minutes. For the secondary exercises, the prescribed number of reps and the corresponding targeted RPE/intensity level is listed.

Quarter 4: On the primary movement (the one listed first), start with a weight with which you can do 12 to15 reps; the objective is to complete 30 reps within five minutes. For the secondary exercises, the prescribed number of reps and the corresponding targeted RPE/intensity level is listed.

While each "quarter" varies in length, remember, you'll perform two exercises. In each *quarter*, the two exercises listed are performed in alternating fashion, until the target number of reps is reached or time expires.

Take a maximum of five minutes between quarters.
For quarter 1, the maximum number of reps permitted on each set is eight. On quarters 2 through 4, it's 10 reps. No matter how good you feel, do not exceed these numbers. Our objective is total workload in the prescribed amount of time.

As a general guideline, most people will do their best by executing the higher rep sets in the beginning, and then over the duration of the quarter, gradually decreasing reps and resting longer as residual fatigue piles up. Think about this as a 15-round boxing match, not a slugfest behind the Persian Fusion restaurant turned peeler bar on Ave de los Azteca in Juarez, Mexico.

Let's take a look at a real-world example. You might begin by performing sets of eight reps with very short (15- to 20-second) rest intervals. But then you start to fatigue, and then you rest longer. Your rest intervals increase as you decrease to sets of four reps, then two reps, and even singles as the time limit approaches. The more often you train this way, the better you will be able to make accurate estimates about your workout.

With the early sets, do not exceed an RPE 8. Some of our test subjects made their best progress by starting with half of what is possible (for example, six reps with a 12-rep max weight) at the beginning of the quarter. But as the quarter comes to a close, you'll find yourself working at or near failure as you attempt to break your rep record, with a goal of never actually missing a weight and never breaking down technically.

So, for instance, on the squat/leg curl example it may look like this:

Set #	Exercises	Weight	Reps	Rest Interval
1	Squat/Leg Curl	300/90	8/6	30 sec
2	Squat/Leg Curl	300/90	7/6	45 sec
3	Squat/Leg Curl	300/90	5/6	40 sec
4	Squat/Leg Curl	300/90	3/6	30 sec
5	Squat/Leg Curl	300/80	2/6	20 sec
6	Squat/Leg Curl	300/80	7/6	75 sec
7	Squat/Leg Curl	300/80	5/6	45 sec
8	Squat/Leg Curl	300/80	5/6	40 sec
9	Squat/Leg Curl	300/80	4/6	30 sec
10	Squat/Leg Curl	300/70	3/6	30 sec
11	Squat/Leg Curl	300/60	1/6	

To hit the targeted 50 reps, it took a total of 11 sets. Rest periods varied based on the hypothetical athlete's needs. The weight remained 300 for squats throughout the duration of the training session. The reps stayed the same on the leg curl, as instructed, but the weight varied because the prescription is an RPE 7. Due to fatigue levels, the exact weight varies.

Progressing

If you do not hit the targeted rep ranges for two consecutive weeks, you need to reduce the starting weight by 10 percent. So, for example, if you were squatting with 300 pounds, reduce the weight to 270 pounds and give it another effort. Each quarter within the workout is progressed separately. You may progress on quarter 1 but have to reduce the weight on quarter 3.

Progression 1: Each time you hit the target number of repetitions, you can increase the total number of repetitions by five and keep the weight the same. You can do this for weeks on end. So, using this methodology for quarter 1 for example (applies to all quarters), it would look like this:

Week 1 – 50 reps
Week 2 – 55 reps
Week 3 – 60 reps

Progression 2: You can also reduce the quarter by 30 seconds, *but* you keep the target reps the same. So, using this methodology for quarter 2 for example (applies to all quarters), it would look like this:

Week 1 – 12:00
Week 2 – 11:30
Week 3 – 11:00

Progression 3: Increase weight. The minimum you can increase a weight is 2.5 pounds; the maximum is 10 percent. So, using this methodology for quarter 3 for example (applies to all quarters), it would look like this:

Week 1 – 155 pounds
Week 2 – 160 pounds
Week 3 – 170 pounds

After achieving the prescribed reps in a quarter, progress using one of these three progressions. Do NOT do two or more. You can literally make progress like this for months.

Lift Execution

For primary core lifts like squats, overhead presses, and Romanian deadlifts, control the negative portion of the rep. On the positive portion of the lift, have the intention to explode the rep as much as possible without sacrificing technique or tightness. We call this movement intention.

Lifting submaximal weights with intention provides many of the maximal weight adaptations that for most are achieved only with maximal triples, doubles, and singles. It also helps with explosive strength adaptations. Your central nervous system and body adapt primarily to this intent and subsequent execution (even if the weight is not moving fast).

Focus on movement intention.

On single-joint movements or isolation movements like cable flys or Zottman curls, the objective is to focus on the muscle doing the work. We call this muscle intention. Put simply, think of it as a natural muscle contraction that happens to carry additional resistance.

Focus on muscle intention.

Movement intention and muscle intention are both very important. We advocate both, while keeping in mind that context is everything. Each has its place.

In regard to the core lifts and isolation movements in the Tactical Density Training program, substitutions are acceptable. While we do recommend following this program exactly, we also realize that injury history and equipment factors are real.

Keep the following guidelines in mind:

- Squats can be substituted for any free weight squat variation and belt squats.
- Bench presses may be substituted for any chest press variation, free weight or machine; the same applies to shoulder presses.
- Any isolation movement can be substituted for another isolation movement that works the same body part.

- Any strongman movement can be substituted for a similar strongman movement.

This is your program. And now that you know the underlying principles, you can adjust to your needs.

The Program
Tactical Density Training comes in two varieties. Choose the program that meets your specific requirements.

If you're looking to harden up before a week on the Gulf Coast, you have a shirtless scene in your local community theater's rendition of *A Streetcar Named Desire*, or you're updating your online dating profile with a more chiseled look, turn to the #Chippendales Ready TDT program.

If you're gearing up for urban combat, preparing for a wildland firefighting season, or just want to stay ready, look to the #GASSTATIONREADY TDT program.

#Chippendales Ready TDT

Day 1
    Squats/Leg Curls (6 reps/RPE 7)
    Cable Flys/Rear Delt Flys (10 reps/RPE 7)
    Overhead Press/Lat Pulldowns (10 reps/RPE 7)
    Zottman Curls/Decline Triceps Extensions (10 reps/RPE 7)

Day 2
    Bench Press/Seal Rows (6 reps/RPE 7)
    Lateral Raises/Pull-Ups (6 reps/RPE 7)
    Dips/Hammer Curls (8 reps/RPE 7)

Leg Press/Kettlebell Swings (8 reps/RPE 7)

Day 3
Romanian Deadlifts/Leg Extensions (15 reps/RPE 7)
Decline Close-Grip Bench Press/Pendlay Rows (5 reps/RPE 7)
Face Pulls/EZ Curls (10 reps/RPE 7)
Chin-Ups/Push-Ups (12 reps/RPE 7)

Gas Station Ready TDT
Unless noted, use the same guidelines as the #Chippendales Ready TDT program.

Day 1
Sled Drags 500 feet/Leg Curls (6 reps/RPE 7)
Farmer's Walks 50 feet/Leg Extensions (20 reps/RPE 7)
Romanian Deadlifts/High Step-Ups (3 reps each leg/RPE 7)
Sandbag Loads/Weighted Planks 15 sec (60% of max weight)
Special Notes
- Sled drags start with a weight you can do one all-out trip with for 70 feet; in 15 minutes you must drag the sled 500 feet. Each time you accomplish this, either take a minute off of the 15 minutes, add 10 percent to the load, or increase the distance by 50 feet within that 15 minutes.
- Farmer's walks start with a weight you can do one all-out trip with for 80 feet; in 12 minutes you must walk 400 feet. Each time you accomplish this, either take 40 seconds off of the 12 minutes, add

10 percent to the load, or increase the distance by 40 feet within that 12 minutes.

Day 2

Bench Press/Seal Rows (5 reps/RPE 7)
Towel Chin-Ups/Dips (8 reps/RPE 7)
Dumbbell Pause Floor Flys/Rear Delt Flys (12 reps/RPE 7)
Decline Dumbbell Triceps Extensions/Incline Dumbbell Curls (8 reps/RPE 7)

Day 3

Squats/GHRs (4 reps/RPE 7)
Trap Bar Deadlifts/Sled Sprints 15 yards (all out)
Neutral-Grip Pull-Ups/Sand Bag Lunges (4 reps each leg/RPE 7)
High Step-Ups/Garhammer Raises (RPE 7)
Sled Sprints: Use 10 to 20 percent of your bodyweight.
High Step-Ups: Aim for a minimum of a quarter of your height.

Day 4

Log Press/Lat Pulldowns (12 reps/RPE 7)
Close-Grip Bench Press/Chest-Supported Incline Dumbbell Rows (9 reps/RPE 7)
Lateral Raises/Towel Kettlebell Curls (15 reps/RPE 7)
Rear Delt Flys/Triceps Pushdowns (15 reps/RPE 7)

Reloading

To gain strength, you can't always be going full-tilt in the gym all the time. Increasingly, you need both "down weeks" and "down workouts." This isn't accomplished by just lying around, however. Rather, you need to plan ahead and include what are known as reload sessions.

A good place to start is three weeks of intense training followed by a lighter week with less volume. Begin your reload week by using about 70 percent of your previous total training volume, dialing back both the number of sets and reps, and if necessary, the weight you use. Some may need to reload more often, like every third week, whereas others can go longer. Your own frequency of reloads depends on a host of individual variables.

Don't use reload weeks as blow-off weeks, though. Instead, use them as *technical reinforcement weeks*. Less total work and lighter weights means this is a prime opportunity to perfect your form.

To start, we recommend reloading every fourth week. If you are feeling good, you can extend your hard training to do a reload every eighth week. However, if you are not recovering sufficiently, consider doing a reload every third week.

Changing Exercises

If you keep making progress on the same exercises, you do not have to change them. You will build a hardened, stronger physique this way.

We recommend sticking to the same exercises for a minimum of four weeks. After this time, you can change, as you see fit, within the substitution guidelines provided.

Neck Work

For the tactical athlete, the neck is the shield. You cannot go into battle without a shield. For the male revue, the neck work is the gateway to the old-school, blood-and-guts, male stripper look.

Either way, you have the green light to do this neck routine up to three days a week.

> Neck Rotations against Band (2 sets of 50 reps)
> Neck Extensions (2 sets of 20 reps)
> Neck Flexions (2 sets of 20 reps)
> Side Necks (2 sets of 15 reps each way)

Active Recovery

On off days you can do less-intensive workouts that span 20 to 45 minutes. The key is to keep your heart rate under 145 beats per minute. These include the following:

- Brisk walking (keep heart rate between 120 to 145 bpm)
- Ruck walks (keep heart rate between 120 to 145 bpm)
- Bodyweight exercises in the RPE 6 range
- Tempo runs of 100 yards (keep heart rate between 120 to 145 bpm)
- Moderate swimming
- Any family or recreational activity

Printed in Great Britain
by Amazon